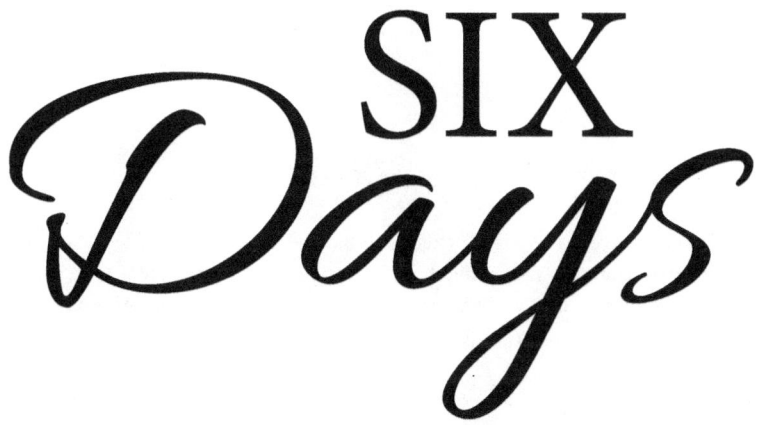

SIX *Days*

THAT'S ALL IT TAKES TO LOSE YOUR FAITH
IN GOD, FAMILY, AND MEDICINE

EMMA RAE

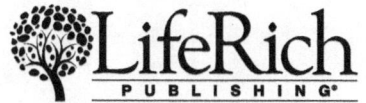

LifeRich Publishing is a registered trademark of The Reader's Digest Association, Inc.

LifeRich Publishing books may be ordered through booksellers or by contacting:

LifeRich Publishing
1663 Liberty Drive
Bloomington, IN 47403
www.liferichpublishing.com
1 (888) 238-8637

ISBN: 978-1-4897-0540-2 (sc)
ISBN: 978-1-4897-0541-9 (e)

Print information available on the last page.

LifeRich Publishing rev. date: 09/11/2015

PROLOGUE

First Do No Harm
Hippocratic Oath: Modern Version

I swear to fulfill, to the best of my ability and judgment, this covenant: I will respect the hard-won scientific gains of those physicians in whose steps I walk, and gladly share such knowledge as is mine with those who are to follow. I will apply, for the benefit of the sick, all measures that are required, avoiding those twin traps of overtreatment and therapeutic nihilism. I will remember that there is to medicine as well as science and that warmth, sympathy, and understanding may outweigh the surgeon's knife or the chemist's drug. I will not be ashamed to say "I know not," nor will I fail to call in my colleagues when the skills of another are needed for a patient's recovery. I will respect the privacy of my patients, for their problems are not disclosed to me that the world may know. Most especially must I tread with care in matters of life and death. If it is given me to save a life, all thanks.

But it may also be within my power to take a life; this awesome responsibility must be faced with great humbleness and awareness of my own frailty. Above all, I must not play at God. I will remember that I do not treat a fever chart, a cancerous growth, but a sick human being, whose illness may affect the person's family and economic stability. My responsibility includes these related problems, if I am to care adequately for the sick. I will prevent disease whenever I can, for prevention is preferable to cure. I will remember that I remain a member of society, with special obligations to all my fellow human beings, those sound of mind and body as well as the infirm. If I do not violate this oath, may I enjoy life and are, respected while I live and remembered with affection thereafter. May to all my fellow human beings, those sound of mind and body as well as the infirm. If I do not violate this oath, may I enjoy life and are, respected while I live and remembered with affection thereafter. Ma I always act so as to preserve the finest traditions of my calling and may I long experience the joy of healing those who seek my help.

Written in 1964 by Louis Lasagna, Academic Dean of
the School of Medicine at Tufts University.

Sam knew she was getting sick when she woke up on Monday morning. By that evening, she felt miserable. She had a high fever, sore throat, coughing, and she was aching all over. She called the clinic to make an appointment first thing Tuesday morning. When she went in to see the first doctor, he told her she probably had the flu and she should go home and rest, drink plenty of fluids, and take Tylenol or Ibuprofen as needed. He did not do an influenza test, which takes about ten minutes. A positive test would have indicated giving her Tamiflu, which is an antiviral medication that decreases the severity of the virus and prevents complications that can arise from the influenza virus. Tamiflu can be given to any patient as long as it is started within the first 48 hours of the onset of symptoms. Sam was seen by the first doctor 24 hours after her first symptoms started. Typically, testing for influenza is recommended when there are a high number of reported influenza cases in the region. The county where Sam lived was ranked as a high number of reported cases of influenza for the two weeks prior to Sam getting sick. Not testing Sam or treating her with Tamiflu was the first mistake.

Wednesday came and she continued to feel awful. She was so eager to get better because she had plans with her friends to go out on the town bar hopping in a bus and she didn't want to miss the party. By Thursday, she was feeling worse. Her temperature was still high and she started vomiting and having dizzy spells. Her mom decided to take her back to the doctor's office in the morning. So, Friday she and Beth went back to the clinic and saw a second physician this time. He noted faint rales when he listened to her lungs but did not order a chest x-ray or any blood tests. He also noted her blood pressure was low. He told her she probably had influenza but did not feel she needed to be tested as it was not going to change her course of treatment. It was too late to give her Tamiflu as the 48 hour window had closed so he sent her home with an antibiotic. That night, she was still vomiting and she started having chest pain.

By Saturday morning, Beth noticed that Sam had swelling around her eyes and she was still vomiting and complaining of chest pain and dizzy spells. Beth was really getting worried so she called the clinic to make an appointment. She spoke with a third doctor, who was the physician on call and explained the six days of her illness. She told him that she had been running a high fever for five days, vomiting for two days, she had puffiness around both her eyes and they felt like they were going to pop out of her head, and she felt like someone was sitting on her chest. The third physician of the group told Beth that she did not need to come in to be seen and these were normal flu symptoms. He said that if Sam was not better by Monday, which was two days away then she should bring her back to the clinic. Beth was supposed to go out of town that evening but was going to cancel because she was worried about her. Sam wouldn't hear of it and told Beth to go and have fun. The dizziness was getting worse and she couldn't stop vomiting. Sam didn't have the energy to keep going to the bathroom so she lay down on the bathroom floor. At 10:00pm, Sam's 17 year old sister Jesse came home to find Sam lying on the bathroom floor. Jesse called her mom and told her that Sam looked really sick and she wanted to take her to the hospital. Beth called her sister Loretta who lived close by and asked her to take Sam to the Emergency Room and Beth headed home.

When my phone rang at 1:30 A.M. and I saw that it was my sister Loretta, my first thought was that something happened to my mom. After all, her emphazema makes her the unhealthiest person in the family. When Loretta said Sam had a heart attack and was being rushed to the University, I jumped out of bed. She explained that she took her to the hospital earlier and her blood pressure dropped after receiving fluids intravenously and the EKG showed a heart attack. I told her I was on my way and I grabbed the nearest clothes I could find. I woke up my thirteen year old daughter Alyssa and told her to get dressed and be ready in three minutes if she wanted to come along. She too jumped out of bed.

Once we were on our way, I called my mom to see what was going on. All my mom knew is that Sam had been sick for six days and they thought she had influenza. Mom didn't know much more than Loretta so I decided to call my other sister Beth. She was riding to the University hospital in the ambulance with Sam. Thankfully she answered but she was still unsure of what was going on. When I found out the Paramedic driving was an old co-worker of mine, I asked to speak to him. James told me that she came in with a high temperature, nausea, vomiting, and dizzy spells. He said they thought she was dehydrated but when they gave her a fluid bolus, her blood pressure crashed (this was due to the stress on her failing heart as it was not strong enough to handle the extra fluid). They did an EKG, which showed signs of a heart attack but they were wondering if she had a pericardial effusion (fluid around the heart).

I couldn't believe what he was telling me and that he was actually talking about my niece. She is only 21 and there is no way this could be right! However, I told my sister that I would be there as soon as I could. She sounded calm on the phone so I was not going to panic. After all, worst case scenario, she would need a pericentesis to remove the fluid around her heart and IV antibiotics. I could only imagine the fit Sam is going to throw at the mention of a needle in her heart. She hates needles! It reminded me of the fit she use to throw when I brushed her hair as a kid. I cannot imagine how freaked out Beth is going to be. They are definitely going to need to give Sam something to sedate her!

When I arrived at the hospital at 2:30am, I found several family members in the waiting room. Nobody had an update and they were all waiting for Beth to give them some information. Beth came out about five minutes later. She said they were just settling her in so I asked if I could go back. Beth said to go ahead and told me that Barry (Beth's ex-husband who adopted the kids) was back there with her.

When I walked in, I was very shocked at what I saw. Sam was lying there on the cot with her hair in her face. When I brushed the hair out of her face, I saw her pale skin and her eyes had puffiness all around them. Why does she have periorbital edema? I told her hi and asked her how she was feeling. She said, "Like crap. Can you make them give me something to drink?" I told her that they probably wanted to wait until they knew for sure what was going on. They probably don't want her to have anything by mouth in case they needed to do any procedures if she did have fluid around her heart. I kissed Sam on the forehead and turned to the nurse. Her blood pressure was still low with a systolic in the 70s and her heart rate was elevated in the 120s. Her oxygen level was 97% which was a good sign. I asked the nurse if I could see the EKG and whatever lab work they had. She did not have anything new but she showed me what was sent from the ER in our hometown. Her EKG looked terrible, showing signs of ischemia (heart damage) in several different leads (showing different places of her heart). Her white blood cell count was not too elevated, which was consistent with a virus. I asked the nurse what the plan was and she said the Cardiologist was coming to do an Echo (an ultrasound of the heart). Since Sam was still vomiting, I asked the nurse when she had medicine last for her nausea/vomiting. She went to check on it and came back with more Zofran (anti-nausea medicine).

Sam was complaining of feeling achy all over and she wanted apple juice. All we could give her was ice chips, which is what we did. Sam would sleep for a few minutes and then wake up vomiting. I was actually surprised how well she was handling feeling so sick but she said she had been like this for days. I felt so bad that I hadn't gone to see her the previous week. I knew she was sick but she had been to the doctors a couple times so I trusted they had things under control. Besides, I had my hands full with my own son who tested positive for Influenza B that same week but he received Tamiflu right away. Beth came back in the room at the same time the Cardiologist arrived to do the Echo. I watched the Echo over his shoulder and could recognize the fluid around her heart. The cardiologist said it wasn't a lot of fluid but he needed to finish the Echo to know for sure what needed to be done. I kept asking questions and got the impression he wanted me to leave him alone so he could do his job. When Beth started asking me to explain to her what was going on, I took her into the bathroom in the room so Sam couldn't hear me. I didn't want to freak her out by talking about needles and such. I explained to Beth that if the fluid around her heart was large enough, they may have to put a needle in there and drain the fluid. How do I explain this to her in words that won't make her panic? These are scary words to anyone, especially the mother of a 21 year old patient! Beth looked scared but stayed calm, which impressed me a lot. I know inside I was freaking out. But all this is manageable and I needed to focus on the medical side of things and not think about the fact that I love that person on that cot.

The cardiologist was still doing the Echo when the nurse brought Sam's lab results for me to review. The cardiologist looked at me quizzical and I explained that I was a nurse and had actually worked at this hospital several years ago in the cardiovascular intensive care unit. This way he knows that he can talk to me like a medical professional and that I am watching him to make sure she was getting the best care that I knew she should get. The nurse asked the cardiologist if he wanted her to start making arrangements for an ICU bed for Sam. He said she could probably go to the regular cardiac floor. I walked out to the hall with the nurse and asked her if she really felt she was well enough to go to the regulary floor and told her I will not be leaving her bedside if she goes on the floor. After all, she is a 21 year old girl! She agreed but reassured me that the cardiologist was great and if he felt she was well enough to go to the floor, and then she trusted him. Well, that was a good sign. He must not be very concerned if he thinks she will be fine on the regular floor vs. an ICU bed. But when the nurse brought me her labs to see, I was shocked. Her troponin (which is an enzyme that is an indicator of heart damage or ischemia) was 0.45. This is the highest I had ever seen in 16 years of nursing, even in patients who had a severe heart attack. It also meant that this didn't just start today as this test has a delayed result and it had to have taken several hours if not days to reach this level by this time. There goes my theory that her doctors had things under control. Why didn't I go see for myself that she was ok? This did not make sense as it showed too much ischemia for a simple pericardial effusion (fluid around the heart). I focused my attention on the cardiologist because there had to be more to the story than this. He was very quiet as he was focusing on the Echo. As I was looking over his shoulder, I noticed the spot where it stated her Ejection Fraction (EF, which is the percent of her heart that is actually working). I asked him what her EF was and he quietly said 25%.

It was at that moment when I separated from being Aunt Laura to the nurse. It was then that I realized how serious this situation was. I have seen 80 year old men with EFs greater than 25% after having a massive heart attack! Sam was critically ill. It doesn't get more critical than this! Beth must have read something on my face because she asked me what that meant. How do I tell her that her baby's heart was barely working? I explained to her that her heart was not working very well right now but also tried to reassure her that she is in the best place and they will figure this out. My head was ready to explode with the reality of what was happening to my baby niece. I needed to get some air so I told Sam and Beth I would be right back.

I went outside and my mom joined me. I knew she followed me out so I could fill her in on what was going on. Everyone relied on me to explain things whenever it came to the medical stuff. I explained to her that her heart was not working very well and my mom was shocked and wanted to know what that meant. I was exhausted just at the thought of what was to come. I wanted to be gentle with her and reassure her but I also needed to get back in there to monitor the situation. I couldn't miss anything medical so I was sure to be on top of everything that was about to happen. I told my mom that she was really sick and that this was very serious.

When I got back in the room, I did my first full assessment of Sam. Her blood pressure was still in the 70s and her heart rate was around

120, oxygen level was still good, skin was pale, cool, and dry. She was continuing to vomit every 10 minutes even though she did not have anything to bring up. She would wake up to ask for ice or her emesis basin but would sleep in between. Her IV was not connected so I asked the nurse if she should be getting fluid. The nurse went to check with the doctor and came back to turn the IV fluid on. She informed me then that Sam was going to be admitted to the CVICU (Cardiovalscular Intensive Care Unit), which is the same unit I used to work in. I cannot believe I am going back there with Sam as a patient. All the patients there were really sick. I started remembering all the people I saw die in that unit or came very close to it. Stop it Laura! You can't think like that, FOCUS!

When they took Sam up to the ICU, we were going to take turns being with her as they only wanted a few people in there at a time. I stayed with her the entire time because I was the medical translator. As part of me was scared to death for Sam, the nurse part was glad because I knew I would be going insane sitting in the waiting room and not knowing what was going on. It is a sense of control to a point, one that I can lean on that the rest of the family did not get to have. I cannot imagine how terrified Beth and everyone else feels, not knowing what things meant or what was to come.

Several residents and interns came in and asked questions as to what lead Sam to this point. Beth was busy talking to them and answering all their questions for the 100th time so I focused on Sam. She was complaining about her back, neck, and legs hurting. She asked me to rub her back so I asked the nurse for some lotion (patients always enjoy a rub with lotion better). While I was rubbing her back and neck, Alyssa (my daughter) came in to see her. I knew she would be feeling scared and uncomfortable so I tried to give her something to do to help and I asked her to rub Sam's feet and legs while I rubbed her back and neck. There we were, the two of us, rubbing Sam. I could see it made Alyssa feel better and I was able to take care of her and Sam at the same time.

The doctors came back less than an hour later. It was probably 8:00 am by then. They told us that they wanted to put in a Swan Ganz catheter (which is a catheter that is threaded directly into her heart and they can do more accurate measurements of pressures and exact heart function) in Sam so they can get a better picture of what was going on with her heart. I remembered all the sick patients that I took care of there that needed a Swan and Sam's level of severity moved up another notch. They must be really concerned if they felt this was necessary. The doctor explained to Beth what exactly it was and why they needed to do it. She looked scared to death. I wondered if she actually realized how serious this was. I tried to act like it was not that big of a deal and that it was what was best for Sam. That seemed to calm her a little (or she was doing a very good job at hiding her fear). When we told Sam what they wanted to do, she said no. She said she just wanted some apple juice and to go home. I explained to her that she was really sick and they needed to do this so they could help her. She finally agreed. Beth was worried about how Sam would handle the procedure so the nurse offered to let me stay with her during the procedure and Beth felt better about it then. I knew what was coming; I could see it in my head. Would I be able to watch them do this to my niece? I knew I didn't have a choice. Beth needed me in there so she knew Sam wasn't alone and I needed to be in there so I knew Sam was ok and I could help to keep her calm and not move when they were putting the catheter in her neck. I asked the nurse to see if she could give Sam something to keep her calm. She talked to the doctor and then gave her Fentenyl to help her rest during the procedure. Sam almost immediately fell asleep. I put on a surgical gown, hat, and mask and they placed a sterile drape over Sam's head and chest. I put my head under the sterile drape and rested it on the pillow with Sam so we were face to face. I put my hand on her forehead so I could stop her from moving her head during the procedure. I reassured her that it will not hurt very much but also stressed the importance of staying still. I explained to her that she will feel a small poke when they numbed the area but she would only feel pressure and movement after that. The meds were working great and she was still sleeping when they got started. Although I had the sterile drape over my head, there was a plastic window around her neck where I could see every move they made. This better not be an intern and he better know what he is doing or I will have to hurt someone. This is not the time to be teaching a newby while my niece is lying here. Stop it Laura, focus on the medical! Sam's eyes were closed the entire time. She grimaced a little when they gave her the local anesthetic but she laid completely still while I watched them take the scalpel and make the incision. I saw her blood start to run down her neck. I stroked her forehead and told her she was doing a great job and how brave she was being. It was like I was two totally different people at that moment. I was Aunt Laura helping her through this and reassuring her yet I watched every move the doctor made while they were placing the Swam catheter into her heart. I could not see the cardiac monitor during the procedure but I knew there was a risk of arrhythmias or the catheter going through her vein or even puncturing her heart. So I watched the nurse's face while she was monitoring Sam's rhythm. So far so good. It's weird as a nurse; I can read the nurse's mind by watching her watch for the same things I would be watching for. It was like I knew everything that was going through her mind, what she was worried about, what she was preparing to do if things went wrong and what the next step was during the procedure.

When everything was done and the nurse was cleaning things up and preparing to get the first readings from the Swan, I went and got Beth to tell her she could come back in. I made sure all the blood was cleaned up as I know that would freak her out. Sam was still sleeping when Beth came back in and I told her how good she did and reassured her that Sam barely flinched in the beginning and slept through the rest. I think that made Beth feel better, at least that was what I was trying to do. While Beth gently talked to Sam and stroked her hair, I was watching the nurse evaluate the readings from the Swan. She looked concerned and focused. I tried to read the results myself but I had to admit that it had been a long time since I had done this and asked the nurse to give me a refresher course on what all the numbers meant. She told me that Sam's cardiac Index was only 0.9, which showed she was in worse heart failure than the ECHO showed. I was trying to process this new information but a voice in my head was screaming, "Are you kidding me? This can't be real. This is a healthy 21 year old girl!"

While we waited for the doctors to give us some more information and a game plan, I called my husband Clay to let him know what was going on. I asked him to come up to the hospital as I knew this was going to be a tough day. I thought maybe he could be here for me since I could not show anyone in the family what was really going on in my head. I had to stay calm and optimistic. If I let them see how freaked out I really was, they would freak out too. I wanted to protect them from the reality and severity of the situation. I told them what they needed to know to get through the situation at hand but sharing with them how dangerous this situation might end up would not help anyone. I knew things were very critical but telling my family made it real. If I kept it in my head, then it was just another day at work but if I told them the possibilities, then it would make it real that Sam was the patient. I could not acknowledge that this was really Sam and keep things together to help Beth and the rest of my family in addition to staying calm to absorb all the medical information that I was going to need to translate. Clay was the only one I could share all my thoughts, fears, and knowledge with about the situation. Plus, I needed him to keep an eye on Alyssa as I needed to focus on Sam and the situation at hand.

The doctors finally came in and explained to Beth that her heart was very weak and was not pumping as well as it needs to. This was the reason for the vomiting as her stomach was not getting the blood flow it needed. The doctors stated that they wanted to put a balloon pump in Sam to give her heart a rest and a chance to recover. There goes that voice again screaming "Are you kidding me?" This is generally done when they are worried that the heart will give out soon because it is too weak to keep going. This is typically the last effort before the heart fails completely. It was at this point that I started thinking about the long term effects of the situation. If she even survived this, there was a good chance she would need a heart transplant. She would be one of those sick and feeble young kids who have to stay in the hospital for months waiting for someone to die so she could live. She was upset about staying in the hospital now and she had only been there for 12 hours! It was really hard to come up with the words to reassure Beth at this point but I kept going. I reiterated to her what the doctors said about giving her heart a break. I told her that this was the best thing for Sam, as it would help her to get the blood to where it needed to go and she could hopefully start to get better.

Her Influenza B test came back positive so at least we knew what was causing this, or at least what started it. If we can give her body some time to recover from this virus, maybe she can start to get better. She may have irreversible damage to her heart, but at least she would survive.

I asked Beth when she had urinated last and she said it was before she went to the ER, over 12 hours ago. I told the nurse I was concerned that she hadn't urinated and after talking to the doctor, they agreed that she needed a Foley catheter because she was too weak to be getting out of bed to use the bathroom. Sam wasn't happy about it but she did agree and the nurse again offered to let me stay with her when they did it. Beth and the others went out to smoke while I held Sam's hand while they put the catheter in her bladder. I thought about making a joke like glancing down at her vajayjay and saying, "Wow, that looks a Lot different since the last time I saw it" (I changed a lot of Sam diapers when she was a baby) but decided not to as she was too sick to appreciate my humor.

When the Foley was in, the nurse got busy getting Sam ready to go to the cath lab to have the balloon pump put in. Things were moving very fast and they were ready to take her back before Beth was back from her smoke break. I called her and told her that they were taking her back and to hurry so she could see her before she goes. The nurse seems very impatient to get going. Does she know something that she is not telling me? There is no time to ask because I recognize the urgency in her behavior and I just want her to take care of Sam. I will ask questions later. I held Sam's hand as they were wheeling her out of the unit and down the hall. Sam had been sleeping most of the time but when I asked the nurse to wait a few more seconds for Beth to get back, Sam looked up at me and said, "It's ok Aunt Laura. Just tell mom that I love her". I kissed her forehead and told her I loved her and let go of the cart to allow the nurse to take her beyond the point that family is allowed to go. Just then the elevator doors opened and I grabbed the cart to stop it and yelled for Beth to run. I could see that the nurse was going to argue with me but changed her mind and let Beth talk to Sam. I do not know what she said to her or what Sam said to her mom. I stood back far enough so I wouldn't hear it because it made my job as the nurse a lot easier (remove the personal part of the situation).

I think that is when Clay and Jake showed up. I took a few minutes to fill him in on what had happened so far. Since the nurse said it would take about 45 minutes to do the procedure, we all went outside to smoke. Clay and the kids stayed in the waiting room. Those 45 minutes felt like hours while we waited for her to come back and everyone was on edge so I moved into my other family role, the entertainer. I'm not sure how my brain comes up with the stuff but it never fails me. I did my best to be funny and keep people from thinking about what was happening.

It seemed like forever but Sam finally came back. Beth, Barry and I went to the unit to see her and she had been placed in another room. Even though the room was bigger, it seemed smaller because of all the equipment and people that were in there. The atmosphere was not like I had expected it. The nurse still looked concerned and when I looked at the monitors, her blood pressure was no better. Sam was asleep but she didn't look good to me so I asked her who I was to make sure she was still with us mentally. She barely opened her eyes but she did whisper, "Aunt Emma". I said good and kissed her on the forehead. While Beth and Barry were at the bed talking to Sam, I talked to one of the interns at the door of her room. I told her that I thought she would be doing better already but it did not look like she was any better since the balloon pump was put in. She said she thought she would be doing better too. I did not say more but I could see the confusion and concern on her face.

I found the heart failure doctor (we called her Jen) in the middle of all the chaos and pulled her aside to try and find out what was going on. I was not feeling good about the scene that I was seeing around Sam. Beth saw me talking to Jen and she left Sam's bedside to come and find out what was going on and Barry followed. As Jen was explaining things to Beth (I honestly wasn't paying attention to what she was saying as I was watching the activity in Sam's room). I heard someone say the word intubation and I went back into the room. I asked the nurse from before what was going on. I could not see Sam's face at this point as there were too many people between us but she told me that her respiratory status was deteriorating and they needed to intubate her to protect her airway. I looked in the nurses eyes and it was like she was talking to me without words. She was telling me that Sam was circling the drain.

I wanted to run to Sam and hold her and beg her to fight harder! But I didn't have time because Beth was watching me like a hawk (it was like I was reading the doctors and nurses faces and my sister was reading mine) and she could tell what was going on. The heart failure doctor was trying to explain to Beth what was happening but Beth was staring at me and I could see it in her eyes that she wanted me to tell her what was happening. I love Beth so much and I wanted to shield her so much but I knew that I couldn't protect her from this so I went to her as a nurse. I explained to her that Sam was not breathing as well as she needs to be so they were going to put a tube in to breath for her. I saw Beth's eyes roll up and her body wanting to give out so I grabbed her arms and looked her in the eyes and told her that it's best to do this now instead of in a situation where they have to. It's to protect her breathing. I think at that point Beth was just taking the information in one moment at a time as her brain could not process more than that. We were standing just outside the room and I was the only one who could see in the room. I couldn't see Sam's head which is good because I did not want to see them put the ET tube (endotrachial tube) in. I saw the nurse make eye contact with me and gave me a nod that it was done. I turned to Beth to tell her they got the tube in and it was done.

It was at this point that I heard the words that will haunt me forever. I heard someone say, "We lost her pulse. I'm starting chest compressions". Is this really happening? This can't be real!!! I turned to Beth and tried to move her away from the door of Sam's room. She was trying to read my face again and asked me what was going on. I could see her begging me with her eyes. I did not know how to say these words to my big sister but I knew she was waiting; pleading for me to tell her what was going on. I took a deep breath and told her they were doing CPR. I could see the panic in her face and she started to run for Sam's room. I grabbed her by the arms to stop her and told her she did not want to go in there. She was pushing against me like a mother who needed to go and pull her baby away from the danger but I knew what was going on in that room and how those images have haunted me even when I did not even know the patient. I did not want Beth to have these images in her head, not now or ever. I begged her not to go in there and told her she did not need to see that. She hesitated for a few seconds that felt like minutes and I could see the internal struggle going on in her mind. She was debating on whether to listen to me or plow me over and run to her baby. I just waited as she was staring me down deciding what to do. Finally she grabbed me by the arms, looked hard into my eyes and said, "Then get your ass in there!' as she pushed me towards the door. I could see out of the corner of my eye that Barry and someone else were taking her out of the unit.

As I started walking into the room, I was waiting for someone to stop me and tell me I couldn't be in there and I was prepared for a fight. I was not going to leave Sam alone during this. But nobody said a word to me as I made my way to the head of her bed and wedged my body between the equipment and the cot. I was taking in the scene around me as I stroked her hair and kissed her forehead. I was telling her to fight harder and not give up. She had so much more to do and she couldn't leave us. We needed her and we loved her SO MUCH! Please Sam, stay with me. You are stronger than this. You can beat this. You do not have all that spunk in you for nothing. Please Sam. I can't let you go. SAMMYMANTHA, you will not leave us! Stay with me baby girl PLEASE! When I was talking to her as Aunt Emma, I was only looking at her face from her eyes up. The other part of me was watching the medical scene in front of me. I heard them say she was in PEA (Pulseless Electrical Activity, which means she has electrical activity going on in her heart but it was not beating). This always has an underlying cause and the only way to reverse it is to fix the cause. I watched them doing chest compressions as they took turns and switched off every few minutes and I thought about how their abs were going to burn tomorrow. I noted all the ACLS (Advanced Cardiac Life Support) meds they were giving her and watched them stop chest compressions every couple minutes to check for a pulse. I felt the same way I always did when we stopped to check for a pulse when I was working on a code (a second of optimism followed by a refocus of what needed to be done). I asked the nurse doing the chest compressions if she thought maybe her pleural effusion had gotten larger (the fluid around her heart. If this fluid had increased, it could be squeezing her heart and not allowing it to beat). She said she didn't know but a few minutes later, someone brought in the Echo machine and checked the fluid level. They said it had not changed. I continued to beg Sam to keep fighting but I could see this scene in my head hundreds of times from my past. Everything we were trying was not working. This was the time we start thinking in our head that we are going to have to stop trying and admit that we could not save the patient. It is at this point in the code that I start thinking of the family and what we are going to say to them. I tried to imagine how I was going to walk out of this room and tell my sister that her baby has died. I cannot think like that. It was at this moment that my brain decided that it wasn't really Sam. This is just a bad dream. A test if you will of how well I can turn that switch and separate from the reality of the situation at hand. I continued to talk to Sam but I wasn't really there. I asked how long we had been going (35 minutes) and was wondering at what point they were going to call it (stop the code and pronounce her dead). I heard them talking about ECMO and I asked what that was. Someone explained to me that it was a heart-lung bypass machine. I asked if that would do any good at this point and they said it will keep her blood flowing and buy her some time. I didn't understand how that would work if she couldn't come back from this code but I just watched and waited.

About ten minutes later, a group of people came and I heard someone say the ECMO team was there. The nurse told me that I would need to leave the room at that time as there was not enough room for them to do what they needed to do. I kissed Sam on the forehead and told her I loved her so much and I was not going to be far away and I promised I would not take my eyes off of her. I went and stood just outside the door in the middle of about ten other people who were watching. There were about ten more people in the room working on Sam. They were still doing chest compressions as the ECMO team prepped her for the procedure. People were running around trying to get supplies and equipment. I heard someone say they needed three units of blood and someone was told to run and get it themselves as they needed it ASAP. I made sure I was not standing in view of the unit door because I was not ready to make eye contact with Beth yet. I still didn't know how I was going to tell her that Sam was gone.

I stood there watching everyone work and I could see people watching me and waiting for me to break down but I was surprisingly calm. I smiled and was polite to whomever I talked to as I kept my eyes on Sam's room (I couldn't see her face which was probably best at that time). I was still not sure what this ECMO was going to do when she was still in PEA. I was trying not to think of the damage that the chest compressions were doing to her, broken ribs, ets.

Eventually the heart failure doctor came and stood by me. She told me that they were almost done putting the tubes in for the ECMO machine and I asked her to explain it to me more. She said they were putting in two large tubes in her femoral artery (the artery in her right groin) and they will be used to circulate her blood through the ECMO machine that acts as her heart and lungs. This will completely bypass her heart and lungs and will provide the oxygen to the rest of her body that her heart would normally do. I asked her if she would still be considered alive and she said yes. She told me that this was the only hospital in the state that even does ECMO on adults. I asked her how long can she be on ECMO. She told me a few weeks at least and this could give Sam's body a chance to recover from the virus. I asked her if her heart will ever be able to function again and she said that we will not know for a while and that only time will tell. I was thinking to myself, "There's no way in hell she will ever regain heart function after this".

They finally told me they were done and the ECMO was working. I asked the heart failure doctor again, "So she is alive?" and she said yes. I told her I needed to go and tell her mom but I wanted to see her first. I went in the room and when I got close enough to see Sam's face, a new reality hit me. Her eyes were halfway open and she had that glassed over gaze that I have seen too many times. It was then that I wondered if we just saved her body but not her brain. Was she down too long? I was picturing her lying there as a vegetable and felt my first pang of guilt. What did we just do to her? Should I have told them to stop? How could I have told them to stop? That was not an option! I kissed her forehead and told her I loved her and was going to talk to her mom but I would be back soon. I left the room but grabbed the nurse that had been with Sam all morning. I told her that I was going out to talk to Sam's mom but if anything changed, she was to call the waiting room and ask for me specifically and I would come back in. I wasn't sure if Beth was ready to come back and see her and definitely not if something more happened. She promised she would and told me they would be moving her to the SICU (Surgical Intensive Care Unit) which had larger rooms and was more equipped to handle the ECMO machine.

I walked out of the unit and found Beth and Barry sitting on the floor just around the corner of the unit. I could see Clay standing in the hallway outside the other unit but couldn't think of him right now as I had to stay focused. I could see this glassed over look on Barb's face, like she checked out while she was waiting. When I told her she was alive, I could see a little life in her eyes. She said, "Really?" and I said yes. I filled her in on what happened about the ECMO machine and what that meant, giving Sam time to let her body recover. I told her she was still critically ill but she was alive. I honestly do not remember if she went back to see her then or not. I do remember that we went out of the unit and I told everyone the same thing I had told Barb and just focused on the fact that she was alive. I didn't tell anyone about my concerns about her brain activity as I thought it was too much for them to handle. They needed to adjust to the situation at hand and we would cross that bridge when we got there. It would not do Beth or anyone else any good to dump this on them after everything that has happened already.

When I got done filling everyone in on the situation, I made sure my other niece Ella and Clay were with Alyssa. I went with all the smokers (Beth, Barry, Mom, etc) outside and told Clay to check on Ella but stay by the phone in the waiting room. I told him to call me on my cell phone if anyone called. I wasn't outside for more than 5 minutes when Clay called and told me to come back right away. I don't remember if I said anything to my family as I took off running but all I could think about was that I had to be there with Sam. If she was going to die, I was not going to let her do it alone. I talked to myself the entire time I was running up there to prepare myself for what was going to happen. When I got to the waiting room, there were a couple doctors in the room. I looked at them and tried to read their face even before they spoke. One of the doctors looked at me and read my face and told me she woke up. "WHAT"? She said Sam just woke up and was pulling at the ET tube and even tried to sit up. "Are you serious?" She said she was and I started crying. I was laughing and crying all at the same time because I knew at that moment she was actually alive. We were still in the ring and we had something to fight for! Beth came up then and she stopped in the hall, frozen in fear as she saw me crying but I quickly told her that Sam woke up. The fear drained out of her face and she looked hopefully towards the doctors. I knew people were looking at me weird as my reaction was greater than any of them understood but I didn't care. She was alive and I didn't just watch them put her through all that for nothing!!! The nurse came out then and pulled me aside while the doctors talked to Beth and the rest of the family. I looked her in the eyes and said, "Are you sure she made purposeful movements" and she smiled at me and said yes. I think she was as shocked and as happy as I was. I can't believe this! Could she really survive that? Just when we get to a point of no return (medically) so to speak, she stays with us. Way to go Sam! I told you that you were stronger than this! I hope she is not mad at me for yelling at her.

I wanted to go and see for myself but the nurse told me they were getting ready to move her and it was going to be a huge endeavor. She told me to make sure I kept the family in the waiting room and showed me which direction they would be going. She didn't think the family should see them moving her as it will probably scare them. I agreed and she told me someone will come and get us to take us to the new waiting room once they got her in the unit.

As we waited for them to move her, I tried to entertain everyone while keeping my eye on the hallway to make sure nobody was in the area when they started moving her. My four year old son Jake was being a monster so and I could tell Clay was getting frustrated with having to chase him around so I told him to go ahead and go home. I don't remember for sure when he did leave but I had him take Alyssa with him. She was very mad at me for making her leave but I knew I would not be able to keep my eye on her and be there for her like I should and I wasn't sure she should see what was happening. She left without saying anything to me, sending me the clear message that she was mad at me. I didn't have time to deal with that so I told her I loved her and let the rest go.

I made sure the family was out of view when they started moving her. I knew right away it was her as there was about 15 people surrounding the bed and they were moving extremely slow down the hallway. I watched them go as I tried to wrap my head around who was in that bed. There was no way that could be Sam.

I don't remember who came and got us to take us to the other waiting room but they told us it would be a while before we could see her so we settled in. I am not sure when Loretta got there but she told me that she had talked to Dad and he wanted me to call him and let him know what was going on. I asked her if he was coming (he lives about a thousand miles away) and she said he didn't know yet. When I called him, the events were starting to wear on me and I didn't have a lot of compassion left, especially for someone who has to even think about whether they should be here or not. If he had seen what his daughter had gone through in the last 18 hours, he would be on a plane right now (or at least he should be). He asked me to tell him what was going on. I asked him if he wanted me to sugar coat it or give it to him straight. He said to just tell him so I did. I said, "Basically she probably has about a 25% chance of surviving and if she does survive, she has about a 90% chance she will need a heart transplant". I wasn't concerned about if this information hurt him as he didn't even know Sam very well. He didn't watch her grow up and she didn't own part of his heart like she did everyone else in this hospital. If she did, he wouldn't be on the phone with me right now. I asked him if he was coming and he said he was not sure but to call him if anything happens. If anything happens? Are you kidding me? I said whatever and ended the conversation. I could not imagine anything keeping me away from my daughter if she was going through something like this.

While we were waiting for her room number to be called overhead to let us know she could have visitors, I finally convinced Beth to lie down and rest. It was 7:00 p.m. Sunday at this point and nobody had slept since Friday night. I encouraged my mom to lie down too but she refused. I took Beth's phone from her as it had been ringing and beeping constantly and I didn't want it to wake her up. I sat on the floor near where she finally fell asleep. I was like a watch dog trying to protect her. I couldn't be in there to watch over Sam so I was going to watch over her mom.

It was about 10:00 p.m. when they finally called her room number. I didn't want to wake Beth as she needed her sleep but I didn't want her to miss seeing Sam since the visiting hours were so restricted in this ICU. Mom, Barry, and I agreed we will go and see if they would let her go back to see her when she woke up. When we went back to her room, things seemed pretty calm. There were two nurses there and they didn't appear stressed at all. Her blood pressure was not great but it was stable. They told us she was sedated so she wouldn't wake up but that was ok because I knew she could and that is all that mattered. While other family members saw Sam, I checked with the nurses to make sure Beth could come back as soon as she woke up no matter what time. They said that was fine and when I got back to the waiting room; I was relieved to see that she was still sleeping. I wasn't sure if letting her sleep was the right idea or if she would be upset when she woke up but I figured she was going to need to rest when she could because who knew when she would be able to sleep again.

Monday

Some people slept while the rest of us sat around talking. I had been up for over 24 hours at this point so I was pretty loose tongued but it worked to keep people entertained. Beth woke up around 3:00 a.m. We immediately reassured her that she could go back and see Sam whenever she wanted, which is why we let her sleep. She seemed fine with that. Beth and some other people went outside to smoke and I decided I would try and sleep for a couple hours. When I lay down, the room was completely quiet and it felt like this fast moving train had just stopped dead in its tracks. It was like a ton of bricks fell on my chest as the events of the last 26 hours came crashing into reality. I couldn't breathe and every time I tried to close my eyes, the images of Sam's code tried to sneak past this armor I had put up around me. I knew I was going to lose it so I ran out of the room and into the hallway. I don't know if I was crying or gasping for air but heard a noise behind me and it was my sister Loretta. She put her hand on my back and for a split second, I didn't feel so alone. I started to let myself feel what had happened and just when I thought it was safe to do so, she walked away. I knelt on the floor of the hallway, trying to get my emotions under control and I knew that when she came back I would fail. But she never came back. I was all alone in the hallway and reality set it that I was going to have to do this on my own strength. I would have to be as strong as everyone needed me to be but I would not have the option of someone being strong for me. So, I picked myself up and went back to work.

I think we all drank about a pot of coffee every eight hours in order to keep going and I don't even remember if we ate anything. We waited for morning to come so we could see Sam again and when we did, nothing had changed. Her blood pressure was still not great but the ECMO machine took away the worry of her heart stopping. That was a relief but there was still so much to worry about. They did another ECHO, which showed that she only had about 10-15% of her heart working at this point. The nurses let me look at her labs and she started to show signs of kidney and liver damage. When I talked to the doctors,

19

they said this could be due to the virus and we would have to wait and see if they would recover. They stated that they may have to start dialysis if her kidneys didn't start working soon. It was at this point that they started talking about a heart transplant. It was also the first contact we had with a social worker. The first time they said the words, I was not surprised but I could see the fear on Beth's face. The heart failure doctor explained that we will have to wait and see if her heart recovers but it would be a good idea to start the paperwork for the transplant just in case. She explained that Sam was too sick for a heart transplant right now anyway but there were several steps before she could be eligible to receive one. We met with the transplant coordinator that morning and Beth filled out paperwork and answered questions.

As the day went on, Sam's labs kept coming back worse and her blood pressure was slowing becoming more unstable. The heart failure doctor along with the cardiovascular surgeon came and talked to us. They explained that her heart was not pumping enough on its own to get all the blood to where it needed to go and they wanted to put a pump in the left side of her heart to help. This would require open heart surgery but it was the only thing left for them to do at this point. I asked them how she was going to be able to get a heart transplant if she was so unstable. They explained that she could stay on the ECMO with the left sided heart pump in for a few weeks until she was stable enough to get an artificial heart. She could live with this artificial heart for up to two years until they found a heart for her. They wanted to put this pump in right away and explained this was the only way to keep her alive and give her body a chance to recover from this virus. Beth agreed and we all sat back to wait, again.

Beth's husband showed up at some point in the evening. I finally lay down in the waiting room and slept for a couple of hours. Sam came out of surgery not long after that. I was anxious to go back and see her and how things went so Beth told me to go find out and come back and let them know what was going on. While I was back with Sam, the orthopedic surgeon came out to the waiting room to talk to Beth. When I came out right after seeing Sam, everyone was upset. Beth was nowhere around (she took off down the hall with her husband behind her) and Barry told me that some doctor had come out and said something about having to cut her legs open and she may need an amputation. WHAT??? I am gone 10 minutes and all hell breaks loose! I tried to understand what they were repeating but it didn't make sense to me. So I went back to talk to the doctor or nurses. They explained to me that when they were bringing Sam back from surgery, someone noticed that her legs felt hard and so they called ortho to come to evaluate her. They realized that she had developed compartment syndrome, which is what happens when swelling in an arm or leg causes the pressure to build up so high that the blood supply is decreased to the affected limb. They explained that they needed to do a fasciotoy, which is where they have to cut her muscles open to relieve the pressure. I asked about the amputation comment and they said that they needed to do the fasciotomy to prevent that. I made sure they were going to have her well sedated and give her pain medication prior and they assured me they would so I headed back to the waiting room to fill everyone in.

I tried to process what was happening as I walked back. It seemed completely impossible that this was really happening. We hadn't gotten over the stress of the heart surgery yet and now we have another crisis? I was trying so hard not to think of the pain Sam must be in. Again, I tried to think of this as a patient at work and not my Sammymantha. I explained to Beth and everyone what I found out and told them we couldn't go back until they were done (I was NOT staying in there for this!).

When we were finally allowed to go back to see Sam, I started my assessment from her feet up. Her toes were purple and cold and I made a note of where the discoloration started and stopped. She had two ten inch incisions on each leg that was hooked to drainage systems. She had four tubes coming from her chest. She had an arterial line in each wrist and she was on the ventilator. They were starting to talk about starting dialysis and eventually decided to start it that night instead of waiting until the morning. I asked if they were worried about her arms as well because they were cool and the nurse said they were watching them. I asked the nurse what the pressures were in her muscles when they did the fasciotomy and he said it was high. I asked him how her muscles looked as far as damage. He explained that they tried to stimulate the muscles to contract (which is a sign that they are still working) and they did not react. He explained that this did not necessarily mean they were damaged because her potassium level was very high and it could be masking a muscle reaction. Once we got back to the waiting room, Beth asked me what that meant. I tried to explain it to her as best I could. I needed to tell her of the possibilities but also keep hope going. As long as there was the slightest chance she could overcome this and all her other set-backs, we needed to keep hope.

I sat back and watched Beth's support system that previously consisted of Barry, Mom, and I get replaced by her husband. I watched her take care of him, even going so far as to make a bed for him while he sat there and watched her. I saw Barry sitting back by himself which broke my heart. Just eight hours ago, he and Beth were helping each other through this, taking turns leaning on each other and seeing the comfort they were both giving each other. It made me sick and all I wanted was for Beth's husband to leave as soon as possible so we could get back to the system that was working so well.

I spent a lot of time in Sam's room that night talking to the nurses while everyone else slept. I was reviewing the labs, her medications she was getting, and brainstorming with them trying to figure out something that we were missing. I spent time on the internet trying to find case studies of similar cases with no luck. I was trying to think of anything I could do to help her. I remembered how easy it was as a healthcare professional to look at a patient as a case and not a person, especially when they were on the ventilator and had so much equipment on them. So I decided that I wanted every person who walked into that room and was involved in her case to know who they were fighting to save. I talked one of the receptionists to let me print off some pictures of Sam and I taped them all over her room, on the cardiac monitor just above her head, on the door, on the bulletin board, etc. I didn't care if it made their job harder to separate the person from the job. This person was a happy and healthy 21 year old girl that was loved by so many people and had a lot of life to live. The nurses finally convinced me to go and lay down and they promised to call me if anything changed while I was gone. I wrote my cell phone number on the board in her room and went to go lay down.

It was 2:30 a.m. and I had only slept two hours since Friday night. I went around the waiting room and made sure everyone was tucked in and then I lay down. I knew that they were going to be doing another ECHO in the morning. As I closed my eyes, I prayed that the ECHO would show that her heart function went up to 25%. I didn't think I was asking too much, considering everything Sam has gone through at this point. I wasn't asking for her not to have this awful virus or that her legs and arms would be ok or that her kidney or liver would start working. I was only asking for 25%. I was not being greedy. At 3:05 a.m., my phone rang and it was the nurse asking me to come back in. He told me that her heart stopped beating completely. I had allowed myself a tiny bit of optimism and God just took that away in less than one hour. It was then that I stopped talking to God. What good was it when he could sit back and watch this happen and not do anything to stop it? If anything, he was just watching it get worse, even when it didn't seem like it could get any worse. It did.

I decided that waking Beth up to tell her this would not change anything and would only take away what little sleep she was getting. It didn't change the course of action, except we knew for sure that her heart was not going to recover from this point and we were definitely looking at an artificial heart. So, I didn't say anything and waited with Sam until Beth woke up and the doctors told her. I felt completely powerless, like I had failed both Sam and Beth. I couldn't protect them from what was coming, a lifetime of limitations IF she even survived. 16 years of nursing experience didn't mean a thing because I could not stop this from happening.

Beth was obviously upset as the reality sunk in that her heart was not going to get better and her daughter will never be the same. The heart failure doctor talked a lot about the artificial heart and that she will be the first person at the University to get one as they just got approved for them. Everyone was exhausted from sleeping what little we could in waiting room chairs so we focused on getting a family room in the hospital. They told us the wait could take days as there were a lot of people waiting as well. This was our third full day at the hospital. As some people left to shower or sleep, other arrived with food. My sister Loretta only spent that second night at the hospital and came up for a few hours a day.

We could only see Sam every few hours at this point and she appeared as stable as she could be. She was not getting better but at least we didn't have to worry about her coding again as the ECMO machine (heart-lung bypass machine) was keeping her circulation going. As we were adjusting to the news of her heart stopping completely and trying to wrap our brain around the artificial heart concept, the doctors came to tell us that the pressure in her arms had increased and they needed to do fasciotomies (cutting them open to relieve the pressure) on them as well. Beth just could not take it anymore and she took off down the hall again. She was sitting on the floor around the corner just staring into space. I wanted to go to Sam but the staff said I had to wait as they were doing it right then. I reminded them to make sure she had pain medicine on board and they assured me they did.

I found Beth still on the floor and when I told her that Tamy, our cousin said it was ok to let her rowdy kids see Sam, Beth jumped up and said, "Hell NO!" Although I didn't want to upset Beth any more than she was already, it was nice to see a little fire in her. It was better than her giving up as she was sitting there on the floor. Beth told Tamy she didn't want any stress around Sam so Tamy backed down but gave me a look and said, "This is not over!" I was so tired and frustrated at this point, I seriously considered going home. Why am I here putting up with this drama, when I could be home with my own family? I mentioned to my mom that maybe it would be best if I went home for a while as I do not want to add to the drama. I didn't want to leave Sam, or Beth for that matter but I knew I couldn't deal with Tamy's messed up family on top of everything else. My mom looked at me with tears in her eyes and said, "Please don't leave me here alone. We need you here". So I stayed.

Loretta showed up later that day and I asked her if she had talked to Dad. She said yes and he said he couldn't come because he had to have a colonoscopy done because he had some medical issues going on. After everything Sam had gone through, not to mention Beth and everyone else, he was using this pathetic excuse?? I asked Beth what she would do if he walked into the waiting room right now and she said she would probably start crying. That was all I needed to hear. If there was anything that could make Beth feel better right now, I was going to make sure it happened. I called our dad and asked him if that is the reason he was not coming. He stated, "Honestly, I saw my doctor today and she said since I haven't had a flu shot, I shouldn't be around there but if anything else happened to let him know and he would come". What else was there to happen? And then it dawned on me. There was one thing that hadn't happened yet. I said to him, "If you are waiting for something to happen, I can give you a list of 20 things that have HAPPENED. How about starting with her heart failing, how about 52 minutes of CPR, how about open heart surgery, how about her arms and legs cut open in ten different places! If you are waiting for something to HAPPEN, you are about 48 hours too late. If you are waiting for her to die, you might as well not bother. Beth won't need you then. She needs you NOW. I love you dad but this is ridiculous!" He said fine and hung up on me.

After that, I spent some time with Sam and the nurses, reviewing her labs. They were steadily getting worse and her kidneys and liver were definitely showing severe damage. She had gained so much fluid because of the inflammatory process and her inability to get rid of fluid. She was actually 50 pounds heavier than where she was admitted. You could hardly recognize her as she was so swollen and puffy. She was already on dialysis but they were not able to remove any extra fluid because her blood pressure was still very low, even with every possible medication they could give her. They had to give her blood constantly just to keep her blood pressure up. Her lungs weren't working anymore at this point either and they were now telling us that her myoglobin level (which is an enzyme that is released when there is muscle damage) is extremely high. This is a problem because it is even more damaging to her kidneys. I was trying to picture her as one of the patients in my dialysis unit and the thought made me nauseous! I was starting to wonder if we were getting to the point where Sam wouldn't want us to continue. The only thing she had left that was working for sure was her brain and I was starting to wonder about that. It had been two days since we have seen any real life from her. Even though she was sedated, I was worried that something had happened to her brain and we would not even notice. I asked the nurses how her neurological assessments have been and they said her pupils were minimally reactive but they did react, which was a good sign. I asked the nurses if they could request a team meeting with the physician and family in the morning. There was so much going on with Sam that I needed to make sure we were all on the same page. Plus, if we were going to have to start talking about Sam not getting better, I did not want to be the one to have that conversation with my sister.

We had to sleep in the waiting room again that night so I rearranged all the furniture to make it look like a living room. I made everyone's bed up and made sure they were all asleep. I couldn't sleep myself so I spent more time on the internet trying to find something that would help us save Sam. I thought about what Sam would want and if she would be happy being completely dependent on someone else for the rest of her life. Would she ever get married? Work? Go party with her friends again? She would never be able to have kids like I dreamed for her. I tried to picture me having a conversation about this and wondered if she would be mad at all we were doing to save her. Then I remembered this video I saw a couple weeks ago about a man who was born with no arms or legs. He goes around to schools and gives inspirational speeches about how he is glad he is alive and how full he thinks his life is. He said he may not be able to hug someone with arms, but he can love them with his heart. I knew then that I couldn't quit trying to save her. I loved her too much and the world would not make sense if she were not here, no matter what condition she was in.

Wednesday

In the morning, I was in Sam's room bright and early so I could catch the heart failure doctor, Jen. I told her to be honest with me and asked her if we were at the point where we need are not doing any good. She reassured me that we were not there yet. She said the ECMO will keep her alive long enough to give us time to see if her other organs are permanently damaged or not. I asked her about her kidney damage caused by her high myoglobin levels and how that was going to affect things. She said she could still have a heart transplant even if her kidneys did not recover. She said we could keep going as long as any one of the three things did not happen: If her liver did not recover (because they cannot do even an artificial heart without a liver and cannot do a liver transplant without a heart), if she had any damage to her brain, or if she lost more than half of a limb. I asked her if they were going to do a head CT to make sure her brain was OK and she said they couldn't at this time because of the ECMO machine but we had no reason to believe there was anything wrong. She said they were going to turn off her sedation today to make sure she could wake up.

I translated all of this to Beth when she woke up and told her we were going to have a family meeting with the lead doctor. I think she was upset and hopeful when I told her what Jen said, as I was. When it was time for the meeting, Beth wanted a few close family members including myself in the meeting. We talked about all the possibilities that Sam was facing. At one point, the doctor said that with so many family members involved, it was a good idea to designate one person to be the primary decision maker in the event of an emergency. Everyone at the table looked at Beth while Beth was looking at me. I told her that I will be here for her to help her understand everything and give her my medical opinion but I did not want to make any decisions. The doctor then stated that it needed to be a parent. Beth had her head down and was crying as she said, "I will do it". It broke my heart to see her like this. I think up until this point, it was necessary for her to rely on me to be this buffer between her and "them" as she was just trying to put one foot in front of the other. But now she had to muster up the strength to do even more, for her daughter.

When we walked out of the room, Beth took off again. We decided to give her some time alone but after about an hour, I started to get worried. Everyone was looking for her and calling her with no luck. I decided to go and check in on Sam and that is where I found her. Something had changed in that short hour. She was talking to Sam and was calm. She had this confidence that I hadn't seen before that surprised me and made me proud. It was as if she knew she had to do this as Sam's mom and she just made the decision and that was that.

When we left the room, Beth said she wanted to talk to everyone that was in the meeting. She said that she did not want anyone else to know the information that Jen (the heart failure doctor) had told us about the three things that would force us to stop everything because she didn't want her other kids, Jesse and Alex to be upset. To keep this information quiet, she did not want anyone telling Loretta because she had a habit of getting information wrong and telling everyone. She also said she didn't want anything negative in that room. She only wanted positive influences near Sam. She wanted people to talk to her and keep things upbeat. (WOW. I was so impressed with her take charge attitude. I was so proud of her!).

At this point, my mom started asking me questions about whether I thought we were torturing Sam by everything we were doing to keep her alive. She didn't think Sam would want to live like this. I admitted to her that the thought had crossed my mind but I couldn't think of giving up yet because that would mean losing Sam. I know that may be selfish but I couldn't even think of a world without her.

That evening the nurses and doctors were talking about starting plasmophoresis, which is a system that filters the blood in an attempt to take out the myoglobin. Sam's level was over 200,000, which was extremely high. There were some issues with whether the physician could do it as this was not a common thing so they decided to do it in the morning.

At one point, Jesse (Sam's seventeen year old sister) was lying on a couch in the waiting room and she said to me, "Aunt Emma, is Sam going to look the same when she comes home?" I sat down beside her and thought about how to respond to this question. How can I tell her that we should be more worried about IF she comes home? She doesn't understand how dangerously close Sam is to not surviving this. I thought about preparing her for this possibility but Beth didn't want the kids to worry so I held back reality from her. "Jesse, Sam is never going to be the same again. She has had a lot of things happen to her body babe". Jesse said, "Well, is she still going to look normal, like pretty?" I said the only thing I could think of, "Sam could never look anything but pretty. Nothing is going to change that. But what we know as normal for Sam is not going to exist anymore. She's going to have a new normal, whatever that may be. The only thing that is going to matter is that she is here with us. I wish I could tell you something different but I can't babe. We just need to support her and be here for her."

We finally got a room that night. Beth's husband finally went back home (thank God!) and Barry went to the hotel to shower and sleep and was coming back in the morning. Beth, Mom, and I were the only ones left. I stressed to the nurses to call my cell phone if anything changed with Sam and the three of us went to sleep around midnight.

I woke up at 4:00 am so I would be in Sam's room before any of the doctors came to do rounds. I wanted to make sure I had a chance to talk to everyone as she had seven different services working with her: cardiovascular, heart failure, orthopedic, infectious disease, cardiac surgery, nephrology, and now endocrinology (her myoglobin level was 800,000 this morning which is the highest the University had ever seen). I spoke with every doctor and felt fairly comfortable that we were covering all our bases. Her hand and feet were still cold and discolored so I spent extra time talking to ortho (her limbs were one of the three deadly sins now). We were all going to go to the cafeteria for lunch since nobody had been eating regularly and I thought a normal sit-at-a-real-table meal would do us all good but then the nurse with the plasmophoresis machine came in. We were going to lunch in the cafeteria when I heard someone mention that this has never been done before. I immediately stopped and said, "WHAT?" They said it has never been done on a patient that was on dialysis and ECMO at the same time but it is a very controlled procedure and if they ran into any problems, they could stop immediately. Her blood pressure was still low and they were still having to give her blood regularly (about 36 units at this point) so I did not feel comfortable leaving her alone so I told everyone else to go and eat lunch and I would stay with Sam.

They brought in this machine and started the procedure while I sat near Sam's bed and read her all the posts she had on her Facebook account. I told her how much everyone loved her and was pulling for her to get better. I wanted to touch her and hold her but it was hard to find a spot on her body that wasn't cut open, poked with some tube or covered with some bandage holding a tube in place. I wondered if she was in pain and I wanted to try and make her feel better in any way. I found a spot on her upper right arm and part of her right hand that I could touch so that is what I did. Her skin was so cold; I wanted her to feel my warmth and to know that someone was here. I held her cold hand and thought of how many patients have commented on how warm my hands were over the years as a nurse, hoping she was thinking that too, wishing I could give some of that to her.

About an hour into the plasmaphoresis, I noticed the nurse's demeanor change. She looked more serious and kept looking at the floor on the other side of Sam's bed. I walked over to see what was going on and there was bright red blood filling one of the chest tube containers. I asked the nurse what was going on and she said she wasn't sure. She left to call the doctor. I immediately started to monitor all the drainage she had coming from all the tubes. They were all bleeding a little more than before but the main bleeding was coming from the chest tubes. When the nurse returned, she said the doctor was coming. Her blood pressure was a little lower than when it started and they were giving her more blood. The nurse didn't say it out loud but I could tell she was worried.

The woman doing the plasmaphoresis said she was done anyway and they were going to check her myoglobin level in four hours to see if it helped. The doctor arrived and explained that when they took the plasma out of her blood and exchanged it with new, it also took out the fibrinogen (which is a clotting factor), which is why she was bleeding. As a fix, they were going to give her platelets to help clot her blood. The problem was that she was already on a blood thinner (Heparin) because they needed to keep her blood thin because of the ECMO so it was a balancing act that at the time, was not doing well.

I stayed in her room for several hours watching her bleeding, monitoring her vital signs, and her lab results. I'm sure Beth was in and out of there but I was too focused on Sam to even remember. Eventually the bleeding slowed down and her blood pressure leveled out. I can't say it was stable because it was never stable. At the four hour mark after the procedure, I asked the nurse to look up the results. Her myoglobin went down to 260,000. That was the first we heard that anything was moving in the right direction. It's funny how easy it was to ignore all the dozens of things that were stacked against us and focus on the one little thing that went right. The nurse said that they were planning on doing the plasmophoresis again tomorrow in hopes of bringing the level down more. I asked if that was a good idea because of the bleeding that happened today. She said that now that they know what will happen, they are going to give her platelets before and during the procedure to prevent it from happening again. I wasn't convinced so I decided to stay close to Sam that night. She was so fragile and things could change at any moment. Her sedation had been turned off all day and we had still not seen any signs of life from her.

Beth, Mom, and Barry must have been worried too because even though we still had the family room, they all decided to sleep in the waiting room again. I didn't sleep much that night. I spent more time on the internet reading every case study I could find but nothing that would help us. I read case studies about plasmophoresis but could not find anything that resembled Sam's case. I walked around the hospital, went on rides in the therapy chair (these chairs that the University has for visitors who have trouble walking the long distances within the hospital). We were all so exhausted physically and mentally that it felt so good just to sit down and be pushed around. So that's what we did. We took turns pushing each other around, we smoked, drank coffee, laughed at anything we could, and we supported each other. The staff had become very relaxed about visiting hours by this point so we could go in the room whenever we wanted. So that's what I did.

Friday

Morning came and the first thing I did when I walked in Sam's room was to touch her feet since it was the closest body part nearest the door. I was completely shocked when I felt her skin warm for the first time since the code. Her toes were still purple but I thought they looked a lighter shade of purple. I then went to her hands. Again they were warm. Are you kidding me???? I wanted to scream and jump up and down with joy. Was this the first sign of life she was showing us? Was she still in this fight?

I was in Sam's room waiting for the physicians to do their rounds. Several physicians came in and rounded at the same time and were talking about their game plan. They decided that it was time to start taking some fluid off of her, slowly and see how she handled it. This was the first time any physician was talking proactively instead of reactively. I wondered if this was another reason to be optimistic but I was still very cautious. I wanted so bad to feel something good and have any amount of hope at this point. Her skin was warm and the doctors were willing to start moving in the direction of recovery!

The ortho doctors came in next. They opened up the dressings on her legs and arms and I watched them do their assessment. I asked them if they thought she had permanent damage to her muscles and he said it was still too early to tell. I decided to lay everything out for this man. After all, he is responsible for making sure one of the deadly sins did not happen. "You know that if she loses even half of a limb, we aren't going to be able to continue until we can get her an artificial heart place. Which basically means your job of keeping her limbs alive is a matter of life and death. I don't mean to put more pressure on you but I am relying on you to protect her arms and legs so I don't have to let my baby niece go." He just stared at me and said "OK". I know I was being harsh, especially to an orthopedic surgeon who isn't used to dealing with this type of life and death situation but I wasn't here to make sure he felt comfortable. I was trying to save Sam's life and if I made anyone feel uncomfortable in the process, so be it.

After all the doctors left, I decided to take Sam's hair out of her ponytail and let if hang loose. It was the only part of her body that wasn't affected. I thought it may be the one thing that felt "normal" to Beth. So I stood there and brushed her hair. It reminded me of when she was little and how she hated her hair brushed but how cute she looked with pigtails. She had a few strands of hair stuck in some tape on her face that was holding her intubation tube in place and I tried to free it. She had fluid oozing from everywhere, even her mouth and I was working hard to keep her face clean. When I tried to get the hair unstuck, I must have pulled too hard and Sam GRIMACED! It was a face that I have seen a million times and I could hear her voice saying, "Aunt Emma, stop it!" I apologized and started kissing her face. I was so happy. She really was in there!!! I immediately went to the waiting room to find Beth. I told her what happened and she almost ran to Sam's room, followed by everyone else.

All morning, we stood around Sam's bed waiting for her to make some movement or show any signs of life. About every half an hour someone would see a grimace and you could feel the hope swelling throughout the room. This was the best anyone felt all week! Her blood pressure was staying just above the danger zone but they still had to give her blood products. The nurses assured me this was fairly normal for someone on ECMO. Her labs were not changing but at least they were not getting worse. I called Clay and asked him to bring the kids to the hospital that evening. I missed them so much as I hadn't been home in almost a week and I had only seen them a couple of times for a few minutes each. Beth and Barry were encouraging me to take some time with my family when they came down and I was planning on going out for supper with them at a real restaurant. They would be here around 6 pm.

Loretta showed up that morning and said she had a surprise for us. Neither Beth nor I had heard from our dad since my last phone conversation with him on Tuesday. I wondered if the surprise was that he was coming. I asked Beth if she thought that was it and she said, "I hope not. At this point, I don't even want him here". I thought about what would happen if he did show up and if Beth would be mad for it. If only I had kept my big mouth shut! I was just trying to stand up for my big sister and it may have backfired on me. Why haven't I learned to just SHUT UP!

I didn't have much time to think about it because that afternoon, they came to do the plasmaphoresis again. I told Beth I would stay with Sam because I wanted to make sure we didn't have a replay of yesterday's bleeding. Although they reassured me that it would not be a problem today because they were going to give her platelets before and during to prevent any bleeding problems, I didn't have a good feeling about it.

The procedure was uneventful but her blood pressure was barely hanging above the danger zone. They were giving her more blood products than earlier in the day (I think we were up to 62 units of blood at this point) and they had to increase her pressors (IV medication that works to keep the blood pressure up). It was about an hour after the procedure was done that I noticed the bleeding coming from her right leg. She had so much blood coming from her incision that the wound vac (drainage system) couldn't keep up and they had to place towels under her leg to catch the blood. She was bleeding from her left leg as well and her feet that were finally warm this morning were now cold again. I asked the nurse if I should be worried about this and she looked worried too and said that they had to give her more and more blood products to keep her blood pressure up. I did not like how this was going and again, I didn't have a good feeling about this. So I went to find the doctor. I found Sam's doctor and told him what was going on. I explained to him that even the nurses were worried. He kind of rolled his eyes and said, "They are just being paranoid because they are not used to having a patient on ECMO, dialysis, AND plasmaphoresis all at the same time. I described all the bleeding and he said that as long as she is on ECMO, we could keep giving her blood products to keep her blood pressure up. I looked him square in the face and asked him if this is something we need to worry about. His response was, "No. As long as she is on the ECMO, everything can be controlled". I asked him to promise me that he will be upfront and honest with me if at any time he thinks we are going to lose her or if we shouldn't continue trying and he agreed and reassured me that things were controllable.

Beth and everyone came back to get me for a cigarette break and mom stayed with Sam. Ella had called then to say she was on her way to the hospital. When we got back to the waiting room after smoking, my heart sunk as my dad was waiting there with his girlfriend and his two sisters. I froze in my tracks and Beth went up to talk to them. All I could think of was if Beth was going to be mad at me for opening up my big mouth to him on the phone. I know that's the only reason he was there and the last thing I wanted to do was add more stress to Beth. Nobody said a word to me (they were obviously mad at me for what I said to him on the phone) so I decided to go back and check on Sam. I had been gone maybe 20 minutes at that point.

When I got to her room, the mood was very different and solemn. The nurse was avoiding eye contact with me so I asked her what had happened. She said that ortho had just been by to check on her arms and legs and all the bleeding. I asked her what they said and she said I needed to get the key players together to talk to the doctor. I asked where the doctor was and she said he didn't want to talk to the family until the heart failure doctor could get here and they were not able to get a hold of her at that time. Loretta and my dad came back to see Sam while I was talking to the nurse and I was still trying to figure out what was wrong. I asked the nurse if ortho was still there so I could talk to them and she said they had left the floor already. I asked her again what they said and she said, "I am so sorry". I asked her what she meant by that and she said that the ortho doctor said that none of Sam's limbs were salvageable. It felt like my reality just blew to tiny little pieces. I knew what that meant. We had just been handed one of the deadly sins that were going to make us stop trying to save her.

I asked the nurse where the doctor was because he needed to talk to Beth. She again said he was waiting for the other doctor (Jen). I became very upset and was yelling at this point, and said, "Go find him and tell him to get his rump out here because I cannot be the one to tell my sister this!" It was at that exact moment Beth came around the corner, just in time to hear what I had said. "Tell me what?" she asked. I didn't know what to say. She must have read my face and she knew something was wrong. She growled at me, demanding that I tell her what was going on. There was not a doctor in sight and the young nurse just stood there like a deer in the headlights. So I told her what the ortho doctor had said.

I could see the reality of the situation register in her mind and she started to collapse, screaming NO! NO! Barry and I grabbed her and she pushed away from us and started to run away. I grabbed her by the arm and said to her, "You cannot run out there right now Beth because Jesse and Alex are just outside that door". She stopped in her tracks and started screaming. Mom came in at that time and saw the scene and asked what happened. I told her what the ortho doctor said and she started to lose it too. Barry and Fred grabbed the two of them and took them out into the hallway.

I turned to the nurse and again told her to go and find the doctor because he needed to talk to Beth. I was so angry at this point. I felt like things were spinning out of control and I was left trying to keep things together. My dad came up to the nurse at this point with Loretta. They had overheard the conversation and he wanted to bring his sisters back to see Sam (they had only met Sam two other times in her life). The nurse looked at me and I turned to my dad and told him now was not a good time. He said, "We just drove two days to see her and they need to come back here". I told him they can later but now we needed to get the doctor in here to talk to Beth and get some things figured out. He yelled at me in the middle of the ICU, "You need to get a life you witch!). Although I was very shocked at what he said, I ignored him and walked away.

I went to check on Beth and found her sitting on the floor in the hallway with her husband beside her and Barry close by. My mom was shaking and crying and Fred (her husband) was beside her. I had to do something as everything was falling apart and I was just standing there watching it happen. So I marched into the doctor's lounge and found Sam's doctor and I told him to get his ars out there and talk to my sister because this is not my job! He said he was willing to go talk to her but would rather wait until Jen got there. I said someone has to go talk to her NOW and I didn't care who it was. He agreed and as he was walking down the hall towards my sister, Jen showed up. He filled her in on what was going on and they both went to talk to Beth.

They took us in a conference room just off the hall. Beth looked comatose and my mom wasn't far off. We knew what was coming and nobody had the strength to even lift up their head while Jen explained that the orthopedic doctor determined that the muscles in her arms and legs were not going to survive and without them, we would not be able to put in an artificial heart. She said we were going to have to let her go.

The doctors left the room at that time to give the family time to process the news and Beth asked me to tell everyone in the waiting room what was going on. I said ok but when I walked into the hall, I couldn't go any further. I was so exhausted and my head was spinning with the events of the last hour. I didn't know if I had it in me to do this. Jen must of recognized my look of despair as she came up to me and told me I didn't have to be the strong one all the time. I said, "Really. Who's going to do it then? Look around!" She looked into the room where my family sat broken and she knew it was the truth. She said, "We can do it together". So she walked down the hall with me towards the waiting room. I got two steps into the waiting room and froze. Jen asked what was wrong. I said, "My thirteen year old daughter is in that room. I don't think I can do this". She said, "Let me do it". I agreed and followed her into the waiting room that was full of about 20 family and friends who loved Sam so much.

I stood slightly behind Jen with my head down as she explained to everyone that there was nothing more we could do and we were going to have to let Sam go. I couldn't make eye contact with anyone because I felt guilty, like I failed not only Sam but everyone in that room. I snapped out of it and back into the nurse mode when I heard Jesse yell, "Aunt Emma!" I immediately went to her and tried to explain what was going on. She didn't understand as she was not expecting it. I felt guilty for not preparing her for this possibility but it was too late now. I found Alex lying on a couch with his head covered and he wouldn't talk to me. I found Ella with her boyfriend and other cousins and Alyssa was with my mom and Clay. My other two kids were there too and they didn't understand what was going on and I didn't have time to talk to them. I gave them a quick hug and called a friend and made arrangements for Clay to meet her halfway so she could take the kids to her house for a while. I heard Loretta say that my dad and aunts were hungry so they were going to a restaurant to eat supper. ARE YOU KIDDING ME????? NOW???? Is she really going to leave me here to deal with this on my own???? It's her sister too! How is he going to support his daughter when he is at Perkins????? I didn't say a word to them and just refocused on what needed to be done.

I told people they could take turns going back there to see Sam and I went to find the doctors. I needed to know what was going to happen next as I knew my family would be coming to me for answers. I asked them what happens next and they said we had two options. The first one was to turn off the ECMO machine and the ventilator. My first reaction was, "No. I don't want my sister to feel like she unplugged her daughter". They explained that the second option was that since she was still bleeding so much, we could just stop giving her blood product. I said, "So basically she would bleed to death" and they said yes. The thought of my baby niece lying there bleeding to death was not an option either. I had to think of something. I couldn't make this go away but I had to find the gentlest way to do this, for Sam and for Beth. I suggested that they talk to Beth but do not use words like turning things off. I suggested they say slowing things down or something like that and they agreed. They said they would give us some time to get everyone in the room. I remembered then that Sam's sedation had been turned off the day before and asked the doctors to turn it back on so she would not be in pain and they agreed. My phone rang then and it was my Aunt Helen. She said Loretta had called her and told her that her niece had died and she wanted to know what was going on. I couldn't even remember if Sam had ever met Aunt Helen or not. I told her I didn't have time to talk right now but would call her tomorrow. Why the hell is Loretta calling everyone and their dog when she should be in here taking care of Beth!!!

I went in the room to tell Beth and the rest of the immediate family who were still in the lounge just off the ICU that the doctors were going to come in and talk to them about what needed to be done and said we should have everyone there that needed to be. Beth wanted to wait until Loretta and dad got back and to see if Sam's ex-boyfriend wanted to be here. While we waited, people can in and out of Sam's room. Everyone was crying and in shock. At one point, Ella came up to me and said, "Aunt Emma, Sam can't die. She just can't. I don't think she believes in God!" My heart stopped and I felt like vomiting right there. I pretended that news didn't bother me and reminded her of Sam's church involvement when she was a kid and that she was baptized. I tried to reassure her best I could but I don't think it did. I walked into the unit and found an empty corner and just fell to the ground, crying. I was only there for a couple of minutes when a nurse came up to me and asked me if she could do anything for me. I pulled myself together and said I was fine and went back to Sam's room. Ella was sitting in a chair in her room crying but it was fairly quiet. I thought this may be my last chance to talk to her alone so I went to her and hugged her as best I could around all the tubes. I whispered in her ear and told her, "I am so proud of you Sammymantha. You have grown up to be such a wonderful and beautiful person. I am so happy that I got to be your aunt. I am sorry that I couldn't save you but I promise I will take care of your mom. You have fought so hard and you have been so strong, but it's ok to let go now if you want". Just as I finished saying the last words, she grimaced. What did that mean? Was she trying to say something to me? Was she scared? Was she in pain? My heart literally broke in a million little pieces at that point but all I could think about is how that would make Beth feel if she saw that. So I went to the nurse and told her I saw her grimace and didn't want anyone else to see that and asked her to turn up her sedation. She agreed and I left the room to go and check on Beth. Should I have gone back to Sam and comforted her? Reassured her that everything was going to be ok? Stayed with her so she wouldn't be scared? But I didn't. I walked away from her because there was still work to do. I had to focus on the task at hand and there was no room for emotions in this situation.

Over an hour later, Loretta and dad's clan finally showed up. I told Beth that they were back and she asked me to go and get Loretta because she wanted her in there when we talked to the doctors. So I did as I was asked. I found Loretta in the hall with the aunts and told her that Beth was asking for her. She said, "No, I am fine out here". I told her that Beth wanted her in there when the doctors came in to talk to us and she said, "I don't need to be in there. I've known all along that she was going to die just like you did". I wasn't sure what she meant by that but I left her in the hallway with my aunt comforting her.

I made sure everyone was in the room and I went to tell the doctors that they were ready. I asked the nurse manager if she could go in the room with them and look out for my sister as I could not be in the room when they talked to her as I didn't think I could keep my emotions at bay if I saw Beth's face when they talked about letting Sam go. She agreed and I went out to smoke. When I got back, Barry told me what the doctors said about turning things down and letting her go. I said that was a good idea. The room was so solemn and I felt like I needed to do something. So I suggested we have everyone come into the room and share happy memories of Sam for a while before we do it and everyone thought that was a good idea.

We gathered everyone in the room. Beth sat at the head of the bed and cradled Sam's head in her arms and spoke quietly into her ear. Ross stood beside Beth while Mike and Barry each held one of Sam's hands. Everyone was quiet for a few minutes so I started things off with a funny story of Sam when she was little. Ella took over after that and it went on like that for about 15 minutes. When people stopped sharing, I quietly worked my way up to Beth to ask her if she was ready but I didn't have to say anything as she said to me, "You can tell them it's time. I told her it was ok to go". I left the room and told the nurse that Beth was ready. I did not look back to the room as I knew if I saw them let her go; the realization of the last six days would come true. I didn't say a word to anyone. I just walked away. It was Friday February 25th, 10:18pm.

EPILOGUE

I stayed to help make all the arrangements and waited until the last person left. I sent Clay home soon after we let Sam go so he could get the kids home. I sent Alyssa home with Ella since she was going to spend the night at my house that night. It was a long and lonely ride home. The funeral was a blur and I do not remember anything that was said. I was still locking myself away so I didn't have to face the reality of what had happened. I went to the cemetery with everyone but when it was time to walk up to the hole they dug for her, I quietly slipped away. Initially, I was just going to walk around a little to catch my breath, but walking away felt so good, I couldn't stop. Running away from this reality is what I had wanted to do since that first night in the hospital. Nobody except for Clay even noticed I was gone, which is what I wanted. I walked all the way back to the church and arrived at the same time everyone got back from the graveside services. I slipped right in with everyone else and nobody had a clue I was still locking myself in my fake reality.

Here I am, almost nine months later still working very hard to keep reality as far away as possible. The people who know me well keep telling me that I have to deal with what happened and start grieving but there are so many reasons why I can't. At first, work was hard to go back to. Walking into a hospital every workday is still a struggle. When a patient vomits, I am worried that they are in heart failure. The blood running through the dialysis tubing sends me right back to Sam's room. I walk into that unit every day and hope with all my might that nobody codes. The thought of being responsible for someone's life send me into a panic attack. I work so hard to keep any emotion locked away and focus on acting normal. People pass me in the hall and ask me how I am and I say, "Good. How are you?" I wonder if they can see in my face that I am lying but they are walking too fast to even see me. On the drive home, I call anyone I can so I don't have to be alone in the quiet car. When I get home, I do my homework or whatever I need to do with the kids.

When all my responsibilities are completed, I make a beeline for my bedroom. I shut the door and turn on the TV. This is the only way I can completely turn it off. I don't have to do anything for anyone while I am in there and I don't have to fake anything. I know I should be out there loving my family, but I can't. I have worked so hard to turn off my emotions; I can't turn them on again. If I do, all the emotions of that week and the nine months since will probably break me completely. If I let myself feel and love, I won't be able to keep these walls up around me and these walls are what has kept me going.

The person that I was before no longer exists. My faith in God is gone. He doesn't love me because if he did, he would have stopped that train from crashing into my life and taking Sam away from me. I have lost my faith in medicine, which has been a love of mine for over 16 years. I have lost my faith in myself as a nurse because I couldn't save Sam or protect my family from this pain. I lost my hope and my happiness and all I have left is the ability to get through the day. All I can focus on is what I need to get done so I can go into my room. It is my cave, a safe place that I can't fail in and nobody expects anything from me in there. I can take those walls that I have built up around me and carry around all day and let them transform into the walls of this room. My safe place where I can avoid the reality of life. I know it is not healthy but I don't care. I don't care about anything outside this room because everything outside represents potential pain and I have had enough of that in this lifetime.

The End

Keep watch for my next book,
The Walls Came Tumbling Down